Copyright © 2014 by Jennifer Greenwald

All rights reserved. No part of this publication may be reproduced, distributed, or transmitted in any form or by any means, including photocopying, recording, or other electronic or mechanical methods, without the prior written permission of the publisher or author, except in the case of brief quotations embodied in critical reviews and certain other noncommercial uses permitted by copyright law. For permission requests, contact the author at www.jennifergreenwald.com.

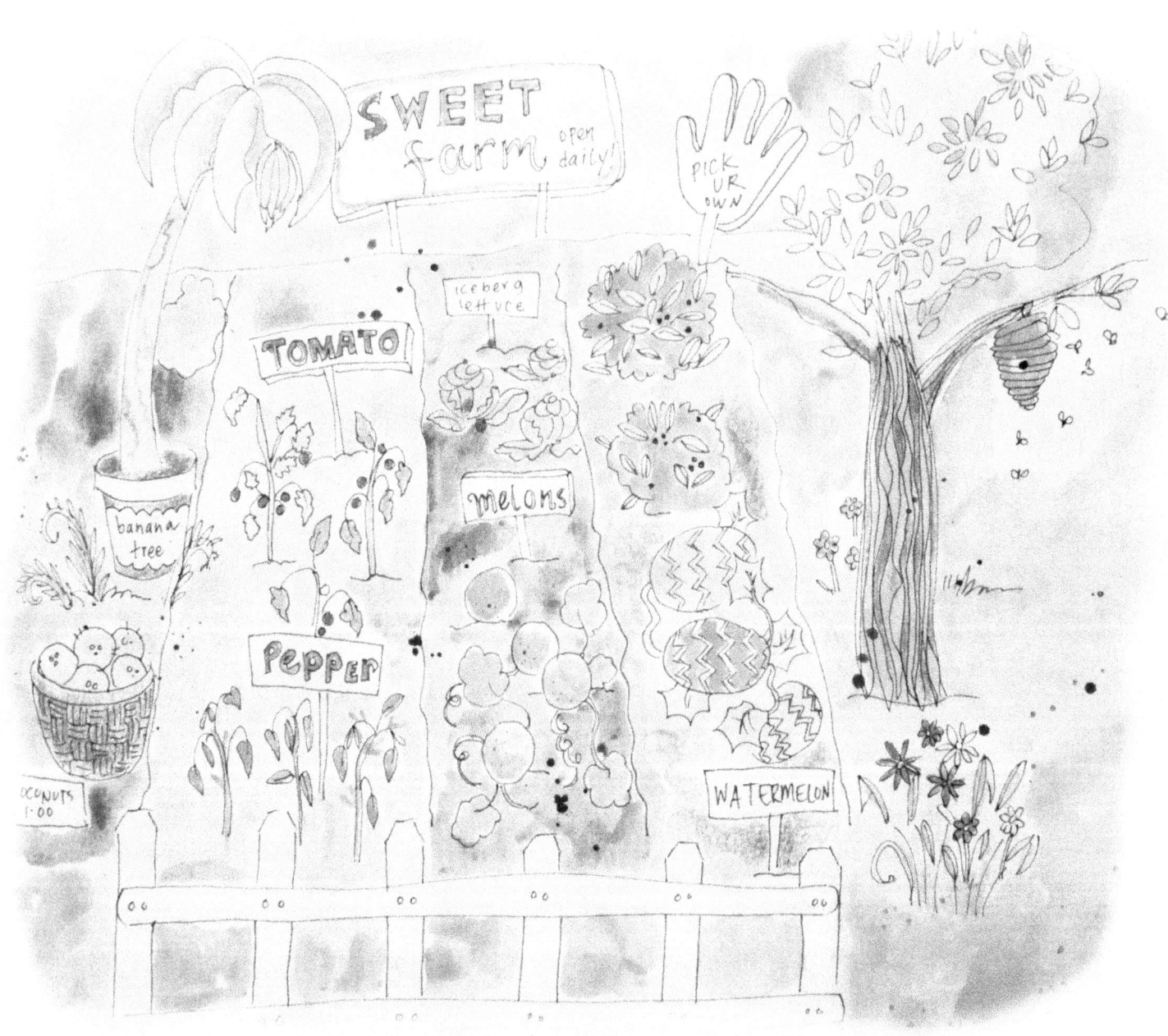

Table of Contents

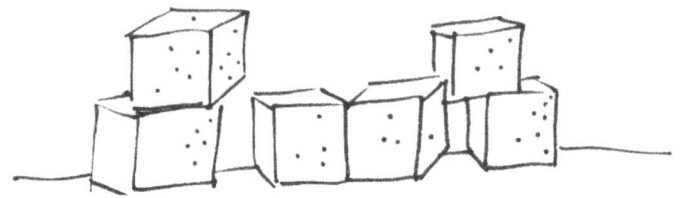

Sweet Challenge 1

Spoonful of Sugar 2-5

Be a Detective 6

Cornucopia Colors 7

Sweet Observation 8

A Fun Food Search 9

Pantry Stick Up 10

Vocabulary 11

Sugar Match 12-13

Recipes That Will Delight Your Sweet Tooth 14-25

Fill Your Plate 26

Introduction

Why This Activity Book?

Have you ever read a really interesting fact and thought you would remember it forever and ever? Have you ever been talking to a friend about that exact fact you thought you would never forget and then, whoops, you couldn't remember it?

Often, we can read a book and get some great information. But then what? You know the saying "if you don't use it, you'll lose it?" It would be terrible if you just moved on and forgot all the healthful and valuable information you learned in *Sweet! The Highs and Lows of Sugar*.

Well, have I got a treat for you! In *Sweet Activities*, you can put your learning into practice! The pages that follow are to deepen your awareness and apply what you know about making choices around the foods that fuel your body. Remember, **personal choice is our birthright.** *We can choose what we eat. We can choose what we think. When we choose well, we live well.*

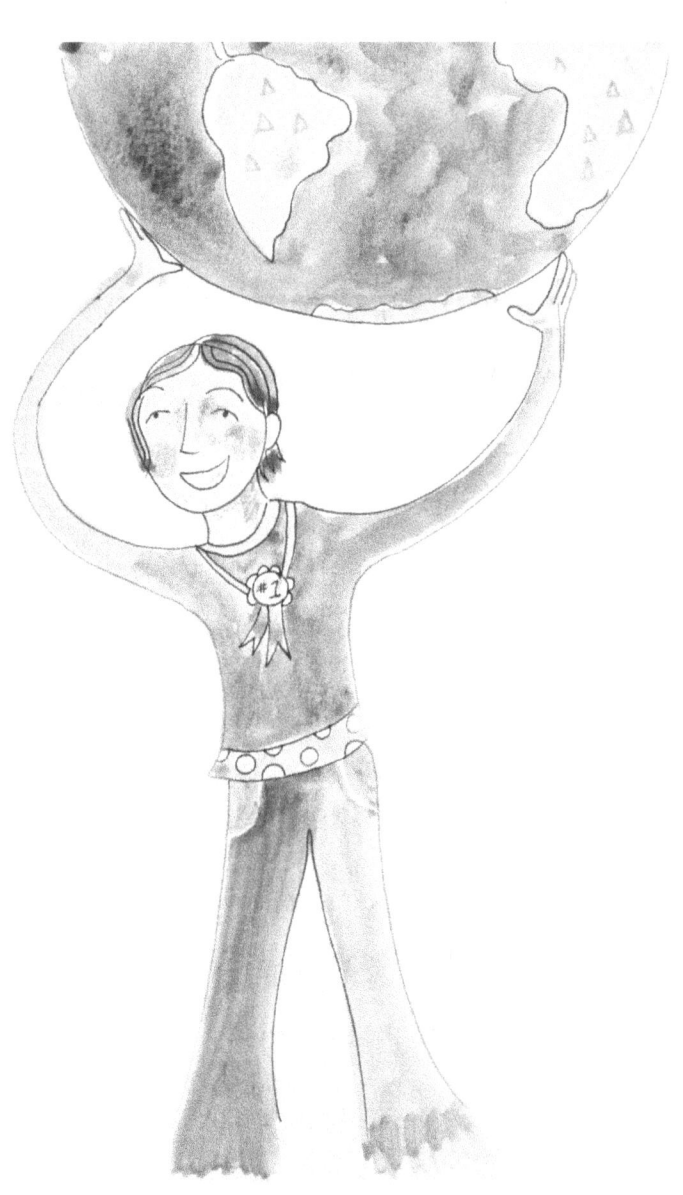

A Sweet Challenge

We can challenge ourselves to eat more whole foods and less processed foods. A challenge can be done on your own, with a friend, or with your family. Either way, make it fun. If you meet the challenge with success, reward yourself with something fun like going to the movies, a new book, or a new toy.

For this challenge, you should try a new **whole food** like a banana, mango, cauliflower, sweet potato ... anything that grows in nature and has not been changed. You also need to eat less of a **processed food**, like the ones that come in a box, bag, container, or bottle with lots of ingredients listed on them.

To start this challenge, first think about some of the foods you enjoy eating. Make a list.

My favorite whole foods: *Whole foods I would like to try:*   *My favorite "fun factory" or processed foods:*

_____   _____   _____
_____   _____   _____
_____   _____   _____
_____   _____   _____
_____   _____   _____
_____   _____   _____

Now that you have some foods to choose from, take one or two foods from either of the whole food lists and make a point to eat them everyday. At the same time, take one food from the "fun factory" food list and remove it for a week.

After you complete the challenge, reflect on how you felt. Was it hard to give up the processed food? Did you enjoy eating the whole food full of nutrients?

Each week challenge yourself with another fun factory food item you would like to eat less and another whole food you would like to eat more. Before you know it you will be eating more and more whole nutritious foods and less processed foods.

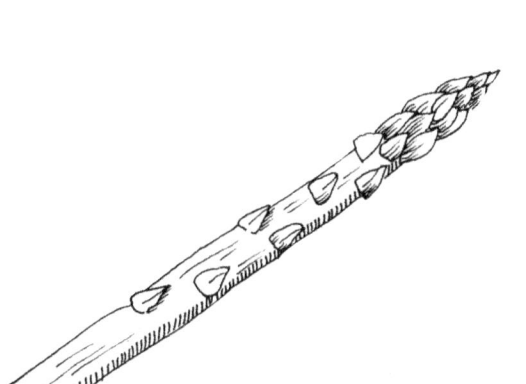
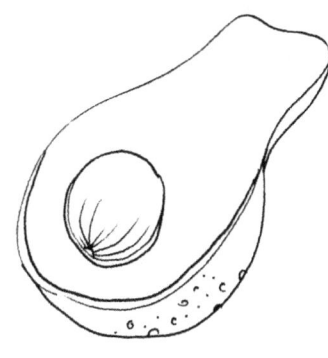

A Spoonful Of Sugar
(refer to page 15 in the book *Sweet!*)

Get to know how much sugar is hanging out in some of the foods you eat.

As we learned in the book Sweet!, roughly 4 grams of sugar equals 1 teaspoon of white table sugar. Generally, you can look for grams of sugar on food labels and divide the grams by 4 to figure out how many teaspoons of sugar is in your food.

So for example if 17 grams of sugar is listed on a label, you would divide 17 by 4 (17÷4 = 4.25) and the answer is 4.25 teaspoons of sugar.

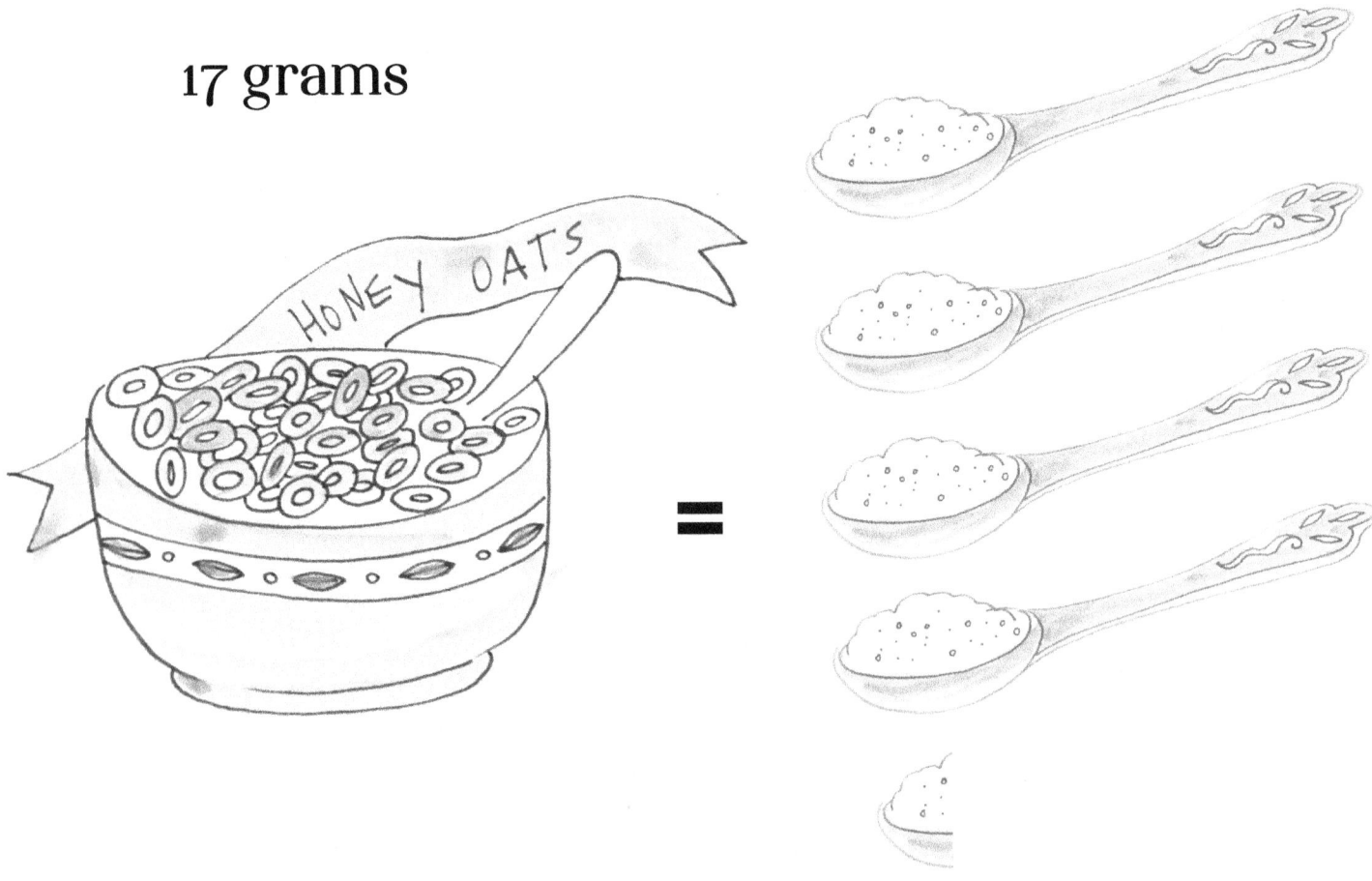

17 grams = 4 1/4 Teaspoons

Time To Be a Sugar Detective!

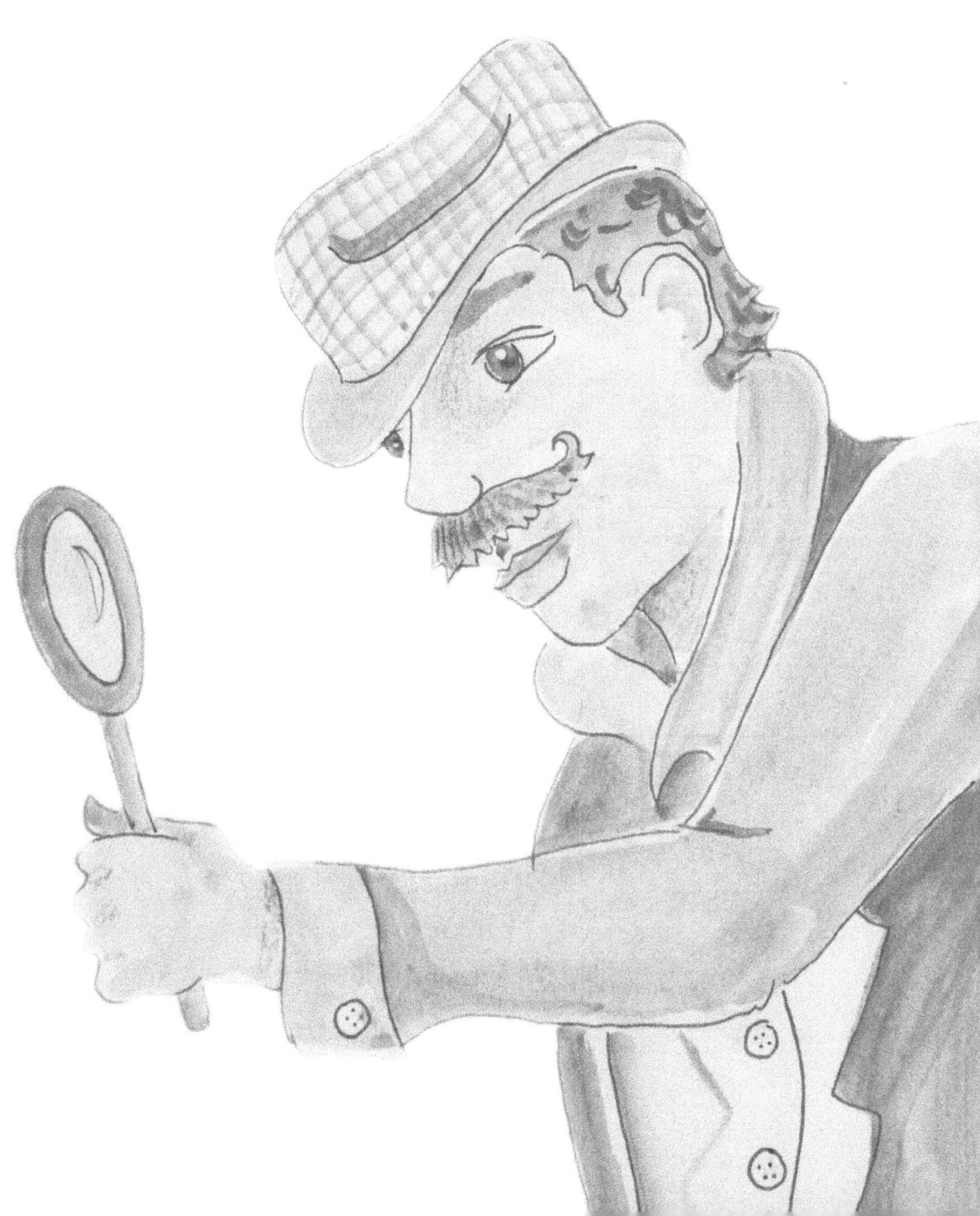

Help Karate Kid Kale find how much sugar is hiding out in these common foods. Write or draw the number of teaspoons of sugar for each food.

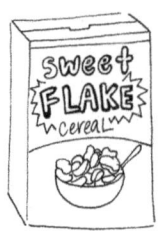
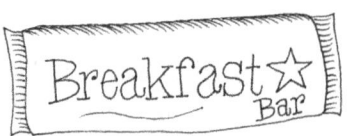
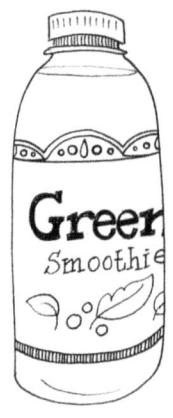

Nutrition Facts
Serving Size 1 container
Amount Per Serving 1
Calories 225 Calories from Fat 0

	% Daily Value*
Total Fat 0g	0%
Saturated Fat 0g	0%
Trans Fat 0g	0%
Cholesterol 0mg	0%
Sodium 320g	14%
Total Carbohydrates 56g	19%
Dietary Fiber 1g	3%
Sugars 21g	
Protien 2g	

INGREDIENTS: Milled corn, cane juice, malt flavor, natural flavor, salt.

Nutrition Facts
Serving Size 1 bar
Amount Per Serving 12
Calories 150 Calories from Fat 45

	% Daily Value*
Total Fat 5g	8%
Saturated Fat 0g	0%
Trans Fat 0g	0%
Cholesterol 0mg	0%
Sodium 60g	4%
Total Carbohydrates 21g	7%
Dietary Fiber 1g	3%
Sugars 13g	
Protien 1g	

INGREDIENTS: Whole grain rolled oats, whole grain rolled wheat, beet sugar, safflower oil, high fructose corn syrup, molasses, dried coconut, cocoa, honey, natural flavors, whey, vanilla.

Nutrition Facts
Serving Size 8 fl oz
Amount Per Serving 2
Calories 220 Calories from Fat 20

	% Daily Value*
Total Fat 2g	4%
Saturated Fat 5g	11%
Trans Fat 0g	0%
Cholesterol 30mg	11%
Sodium 150g	7%
Total Carbohydrates 31g	7%
Dietary Fiber 0g	0%
Sugars 28g	
Protien 17g	

INGREDIENTS: Apple juice, puree banana, pineapple juice, orange juice, honey, whey protein, soy protein, coconut milk, natural flavors

_____   _____   _____

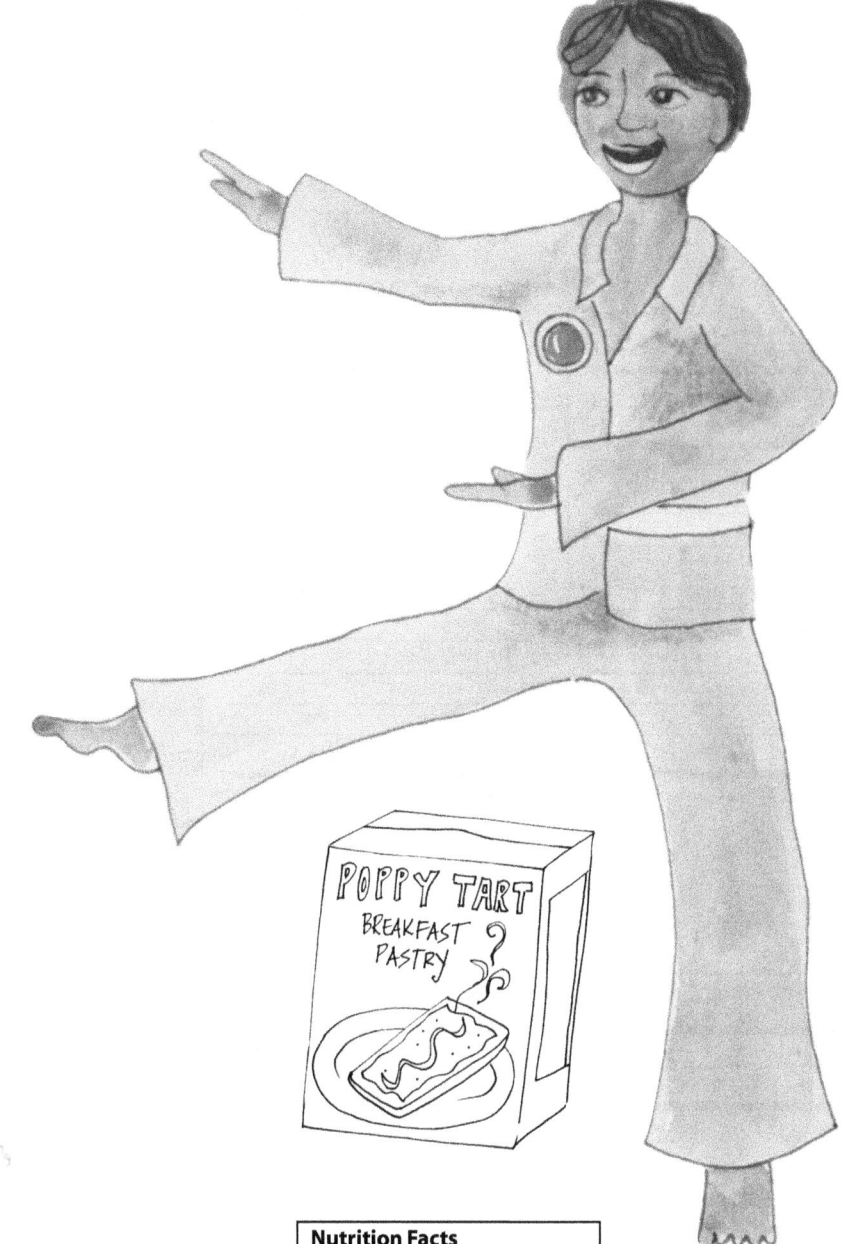

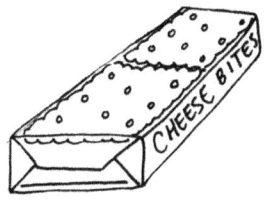

Nutrition Facts
Serving Size 1 package

Amount Per Serving 8

Calories 210   Calories from Fat 95

	% Daily Value*
Total Fat 10g	16%
Saturated Fat 2.5g	13%
Trans Fat 0g	0%
Cholesterol 0mg	0%
Sodium 300g	12%
Total Carbohydrates 21g	7%
Dietary Fiber 1g	3%
Sugars 5g	
Protien 3g	

INGREDIENTS: Enriched flour, vegetable oil, whey, inverted cane sugar, cheddar cheese, milk, butter, natural and artificial flavors, yellow #6, turmeric, red pepper.

_____

Nutrition Facts
Serving Size 1 pastry

Amount Per Serving 8

Calories 190   Calories from Fat 40

	% Daily Value*
Total Fat 6g	9%
Saturated Fat 2g	9%
Trans Fat 0g	0%
Cholesterol 0mg	0%
Sodium 180g	7%
Total Carbohydrates 36g	12%
Dietary Fiber 1g	3%
Sugars 16g	
Protien 2g	

INGREDIENTS: Enriched flour, brown rice syrup, high fructose corn syrup, dextrose, palm oil, salt, dried blueberries, dried grapes, dried apples, baking soda, citric acid.

_____

Be A Detective

(refer to page 12 in the book *Sweet!*)

Sugar loves to hide in food and it's your job to be a food detective. Help Sweet Maple by using your detective skills to read these labels and find the hidden sugars. Some foods have more then one!!

Nutrition Facts
Serving Size 1 muffin
Amount Per Serving 12
Calories 200   Calories from Fat 70

	% Daily Value*
Total Fat 8g	12%
Saturated Fat 1.5g	8%
Trans Fat 0g	0%
Cholesterol 35g	12%
Sodium 200g	8%
Total Carbohydrates 30g	10%
Dietary Fiber 3g	12%
Sugars 15g	
Protien 3g	

INGREDIENTS: Whole wheat flour, wheat flour, cane sugar, palm oil, dextrose, dextrin, corn starch, baking powder, natural flavor, salt, xanthan, and guar gum.

Nutrition Facts
Serving Size 4 crackers
Amount Per Serving 10
Calories 70   Calories from Fat 20

	% Daily Value*
Total Fat 2g	3%
Saturated Fat 0g	0%
Trans Fat 0g	0%
Cholesterol 0mg	0%
Sodium 160g	7%
Total Carbohydrates 12g	4%
Dietary Fiber 0g	0%
Sugars 3g	
Protien 1g	

INGREDIENTS: Organic wheat flour, organic evaporated cane juice, organic pressed sunflower oil, organic palm oil, baking soda, cream of tartar, xantham, salt.

Nutrition Facts
Serving Size 4 cookies
Amount Per Serving 4
Calories 260   Calories from Fat 105

	% Daily Value*
Total Fat 13g	18%
Saturated Fat 6g	36%
Trans Fat 0g	0%
Cholesterol 35mg	15%
Sodium 160g	7%
Total Carbohydrates 36g	13%
Dietary Fiber 2g	3%
Sugars 23g	
Protien 2g	

INGREDIENTS: Rice flour, tapioca, turbinado, cocoa butter, soy lecithin, vanilla, sugar in the raw, butter, eggs, unsulphured molasses, potato starch, corn starch, salt, baking soda.

Nutrition Facts
Serving Size 1 Tablespoon
Amount Per Serving 20
Calories 50   Calories from Fat 0

	% Daily Value*
Total Fat 0g	0%
Saturated Fat 0g	0%
Trans Fat 0g	0%
Cholesterol 0mg	0%
Sodium 0g	0%
Total Carbohydrates 12g	4%
Dietary Fiber 0g	0%
Sugars 12g	
Protien 0g	

INGREDIENTS: Raspberries, corn syrup, fruit pectin, orange juice, lemon concentrate

Nutrition Facts
Serving Size 4 pieces
Amount Per Serving 8
Calories 230   Calories from Fat 120

	% Daily Value*
Total Fat 13g	20%
Saturated Fat 5g	25%
Trans Fat 0g	0%
Cholesterol 13mg	6%
Sodium 155g	6%
Total Carbohydrates 27g	9%
Dietary Fiber 0g	0%
Sugars 17g	
Protien 3g	

INGREDIENTS: Enriched flour, water, palm oil, soybean oil, egg yolks, baking soda, aluminum phosphate, soy flour, whey, corn syrup solids, high fructose corn syrup, salt, wheat, starch, brown rice syrup, polysorbate, xanthan gum, nutmeg oil, wheat

Nutrition Facts
Serving Size 1 patty
Amount Per Serving 4
Calories 180   Calories from Fat 15

	% Daily Value*
Total Fat 2g	4%
Saturated Fat 0g	0%
Trans Fat 0g	0%
Cholesterol 0mg	0%
Sodium 300g	14%
Total Carbohydrates 27g	12%
Dietary Fiber 2g	3%
Sugars 2g	
Protien 8g	

INGREDIENTS: Water, soy protein, cheddar cheese, onions, carmel color, beet juice, whey, brown rice syrup, spices and herbs, yeast extract.

Now that you have some practice being a detective, take your detective skills with you to the grocery store and to your pantry when you are hungry for something to eat.

Cornucopia Colors

Sweet Maple and Karate Kid Kale love trying new foods and flavors. What foods have you tried on this page? Color the whole foods you have eaten at least once in your life. Notice the foods you have not tried. Color them in as you try them. Over time, the goal is to have colored the entire cornucopia!

Look how colorful the cornucopia is once you have it completed. Eating a variety of colors (natural whole food colors!) is a sure way to stay healthy! Bon Appetite!

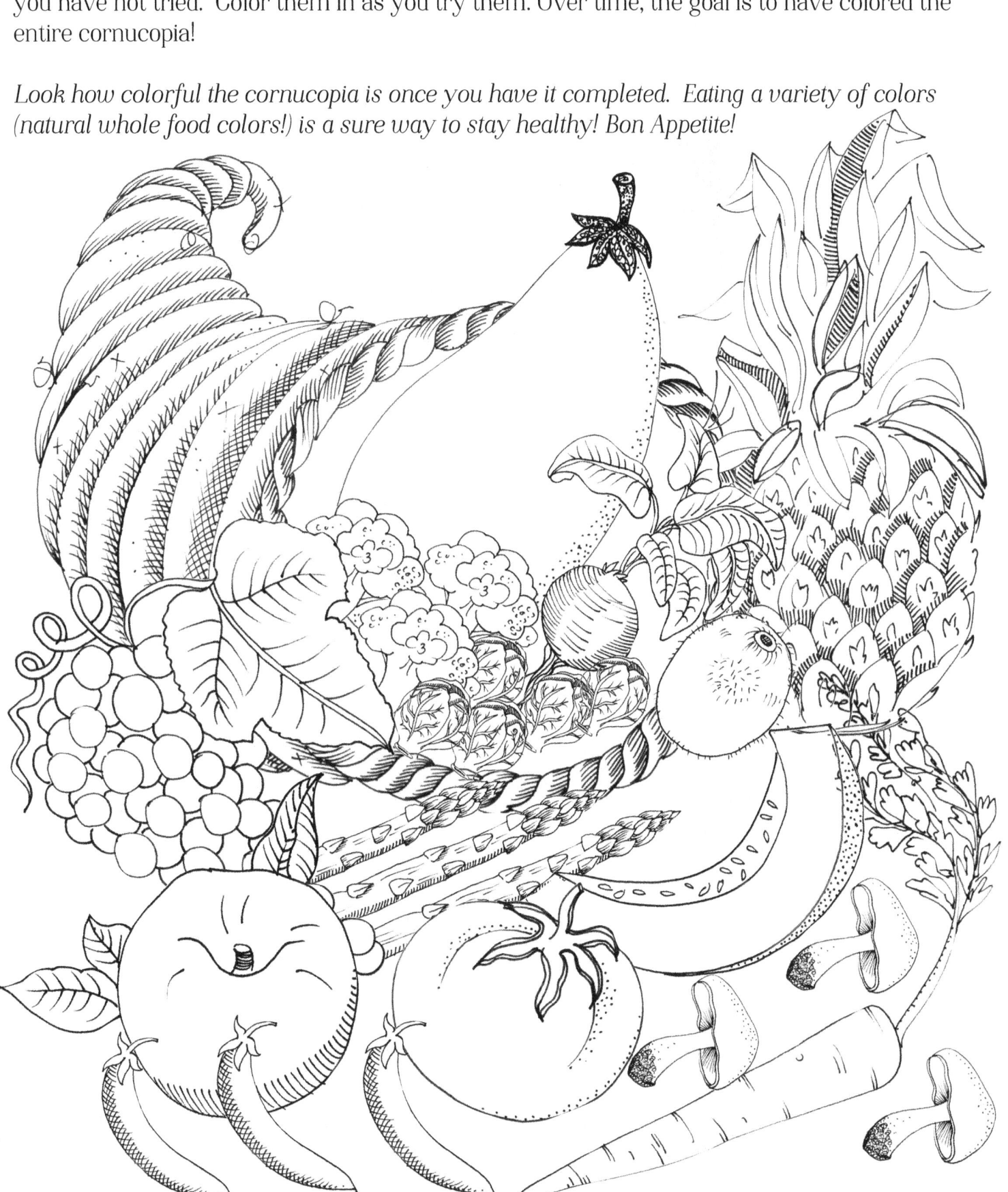

Sweet Observation

Eat a cupcake or a candy bar or a bag of chips. Yep! I just gave you permission to eat some processed junk food! (You must also get permission from your parents.) Here is the catch! Before you eat it, you need to agree to do an observation.

When you eat your choice of processed junk food, notice how you are feeling as you eat. Bring your senses to the eating experience. What does your food look like? How does it smell? What flavors do you taste?

Now wait about 30 minutes and notice how you are feeling again. Are you hungry? Do you feel tired? Did you have a burst of energy followed by a crash? Discuss your observation with a friend or family member.

Sweet Maple and Karate Kid Kale would like you to try something else. Do the same experiment eating whole foods. What do you notice?

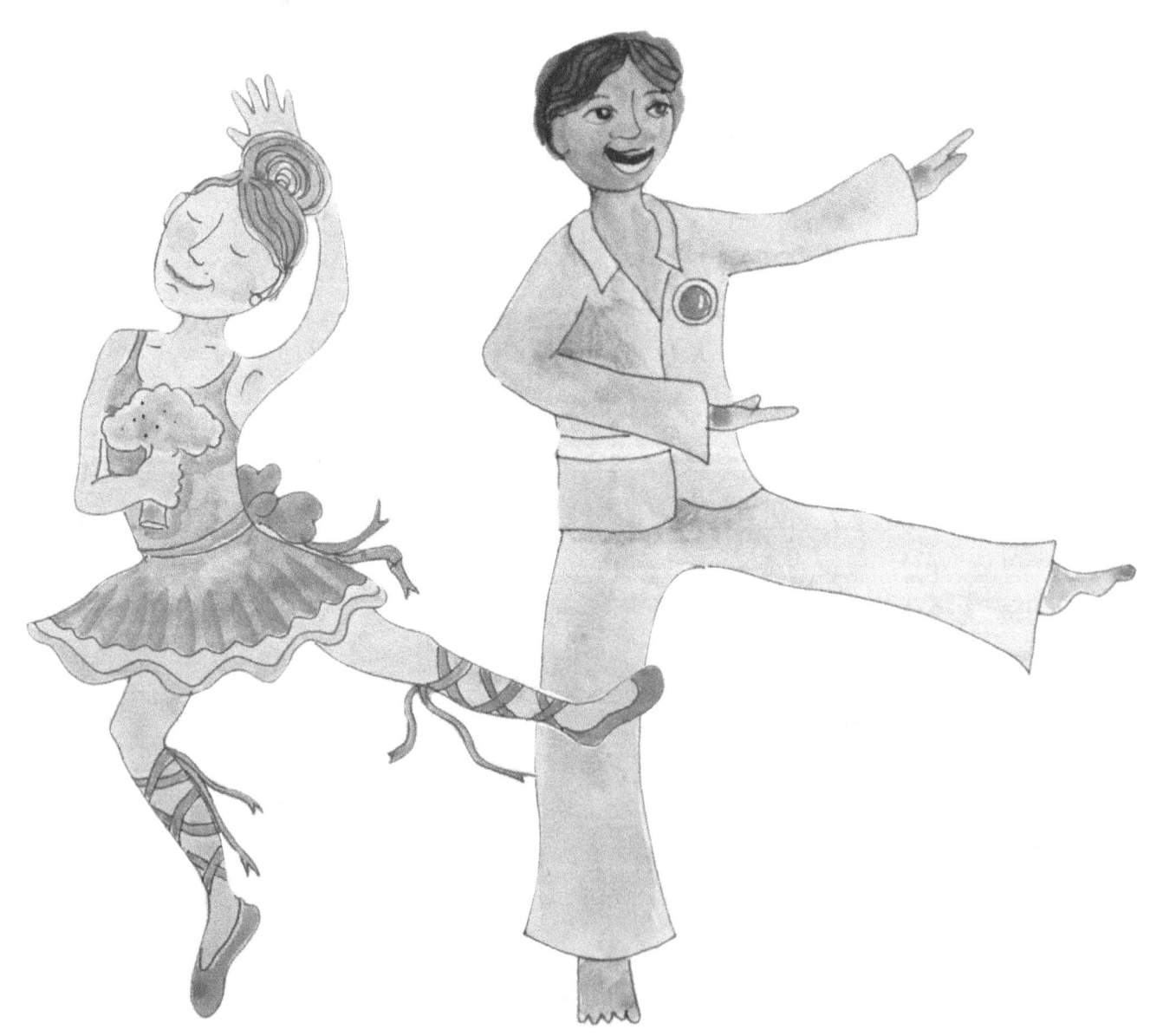

A Fun Food Search

You will need to use your detective skills for this activity. Find the following foods in the word search. Circle the whole foods in green. Circle the processed foods in purple.

grapes	apple	avocado	cereal bar
chips	potato	soda	bagel
honey	crackers	cookie	
lollipop	melon	carrot	

```
c  t  m  b  c  k  c  b  l  s  g  r  a  t  w  r  t  l  p
f  r  c  a  r  r  h  o  p  f  r  u  i  t  s  n  a  c  k
p  c  i  l  a  p  i  m  t  r  a  f  n  l  o  r  d  r  a
h  e  p  g  r  a  p  e  s  o  p  l  b  c  l  h  d  a  y
n  r  e  n  k  i  s  p  o  l  p  o  t  a  t  o  m  c  c
b  e  m  p  r  a  p  f  d  t  o  n  e  r  b  n  o  k  o
f  a  m  i  d  p  o  d  a  l  b  a  n  r  d  e  a  e  o
a  l  e  w  g  p  t  s  p  i  m  b  l  o  t  y  l  r  k
c  b  l  l  o  l  l  i  p  o  p  e  a  t  v  l  i  s  i
u  a  o  e  n  e  s  p  l  r  e  t  y  u  f  m  s  n  e
l  r  n  p  r  d  b  a  g  e  l  a  v  o  c  a  d  o  d
```

Pantry Stick Up

(refer to page 12 in the book *Sweet!*)

Materials Needed:
Green dot stickers and red dot stickers

Karate Kid Kale and Sweet Maple love knowing which foods are nourishing to eat. One way you can do this is to look through your pantry. Read the ingredients on the labels. Place a red dot sticker on the foods with sneaky processed sugars. Place a green dot on the foods with natural, whole sources of sugars. Some items may have both!!

How many green dots are in your pantry?

How many red dots are in your pantry?

What did you notice? Which color stickers did you use the most?
Do you eat a lot of foods with added sugar? Or are most of the foods you eat whole foods? Have a family discussion about your realizations.

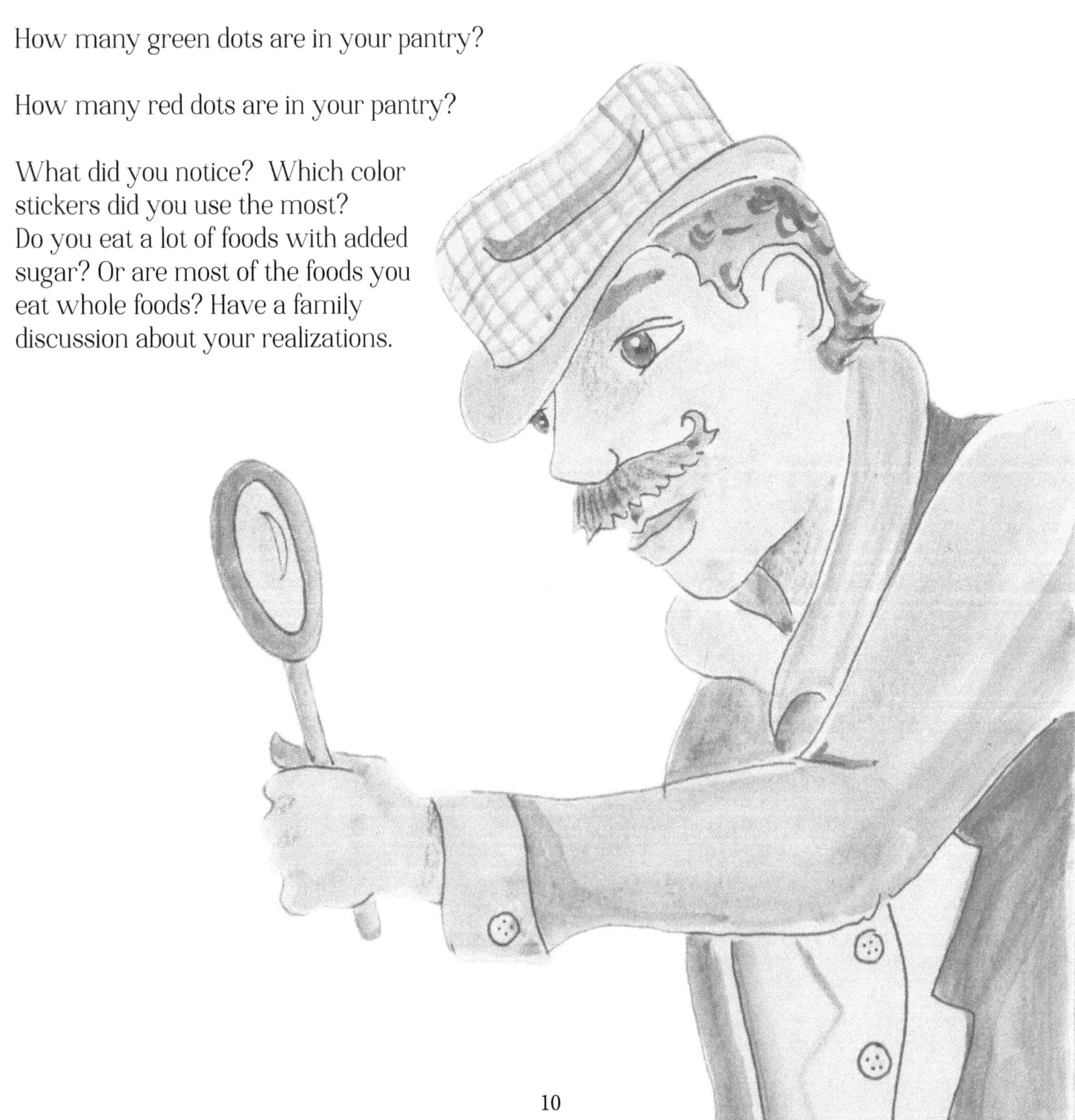

Vocabulary

On page 12 in the book *Sweet!* some common names for sugar are listed. These are not the only names for sugar. There are even more! What other names for sugar can you find that are not listed in the book?

You may have to use a computer and begin a search to find other names used for sugar. How many more can you find?

_____	_____	_____
_____	_____	_____
_____	_____	_____
_____	_____	_____
_____	_____	_____
_____	_____	_____

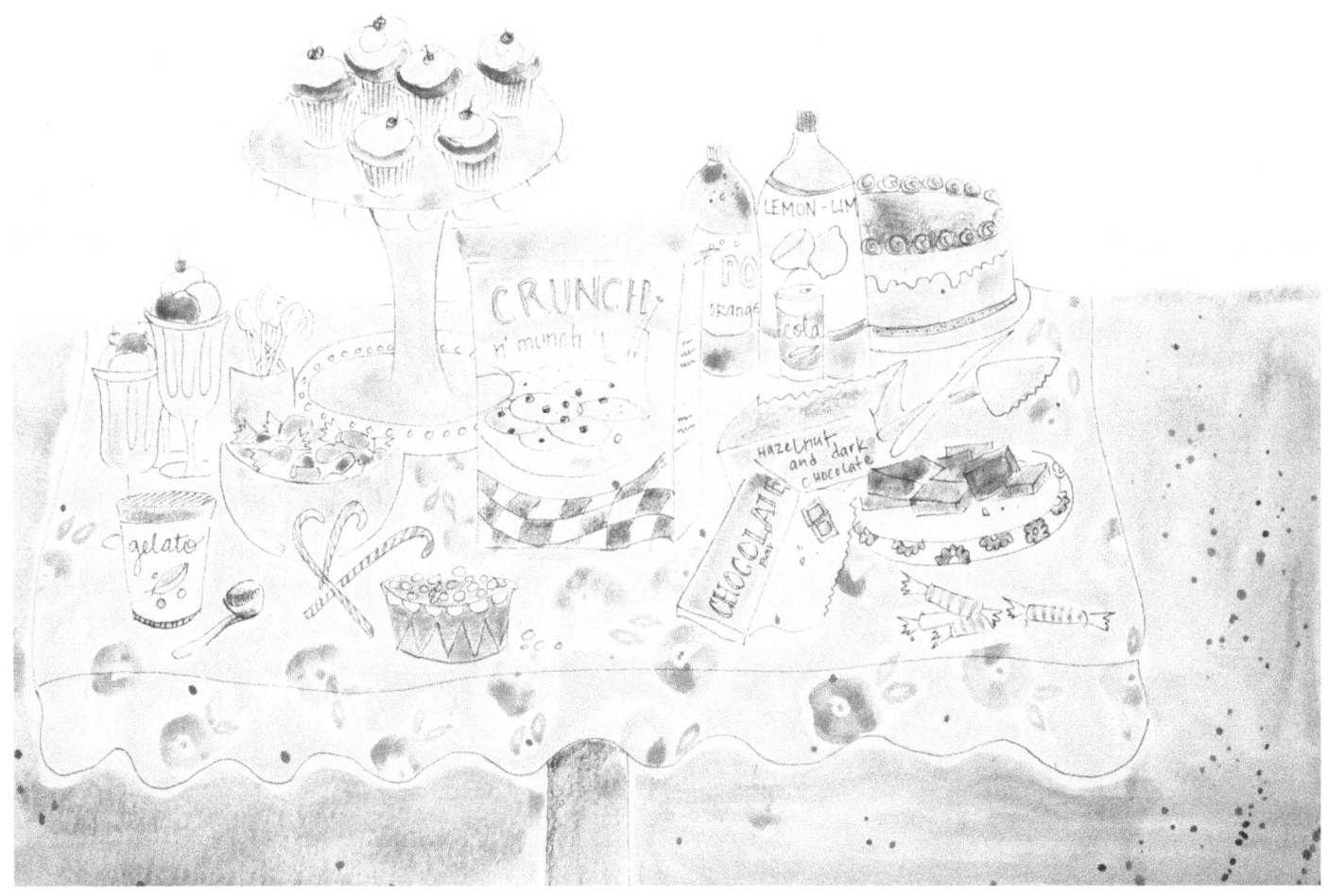

Sugar Match

Help Sweet Maple match each source of sugar below to how it is seen growing in nature. The foods are marked with letters. Match the letters to their source on the following page. Write your answer on the blank line.

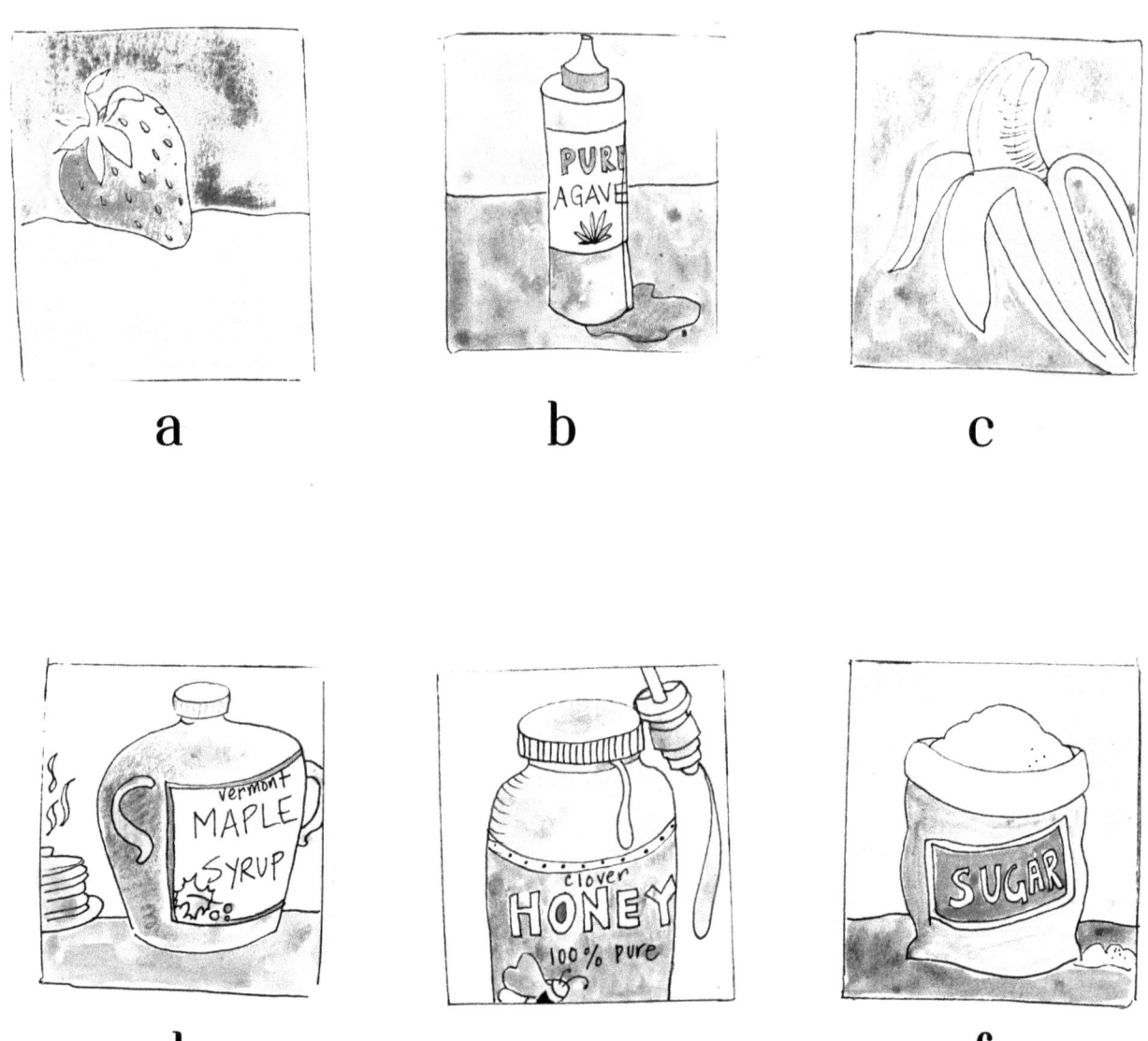

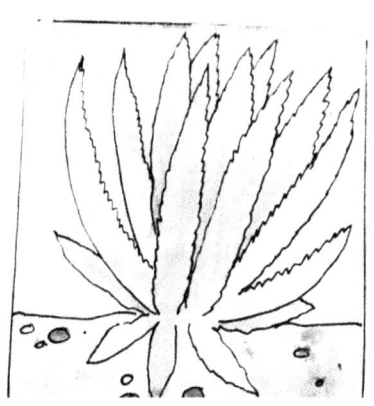
_____

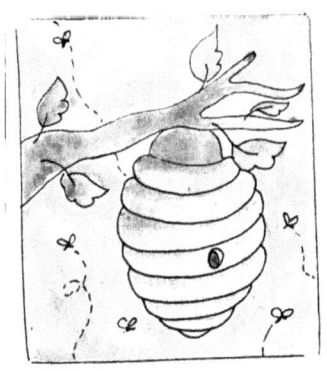
_____

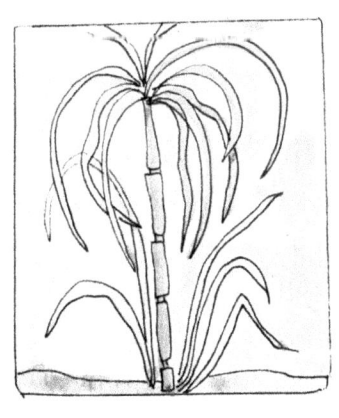
_____

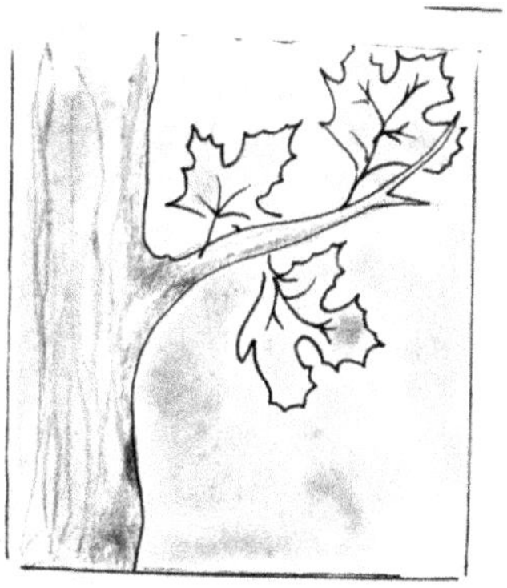

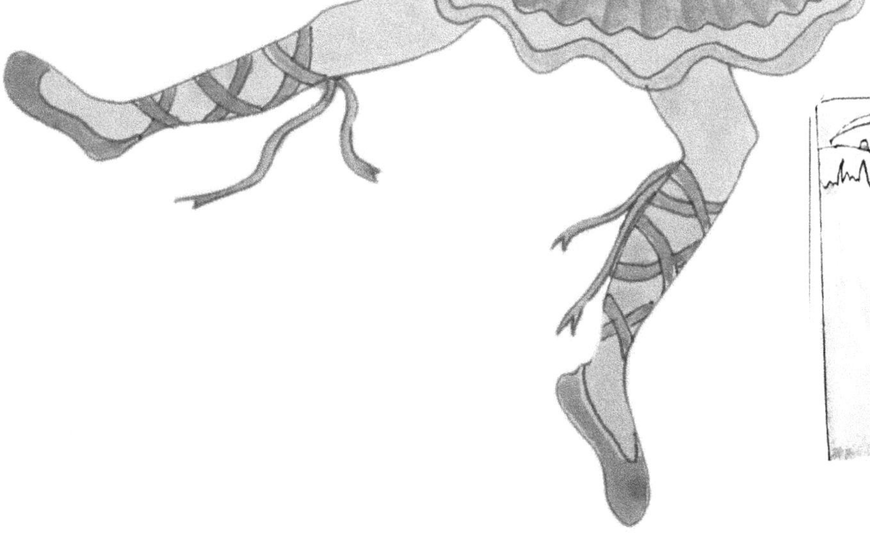

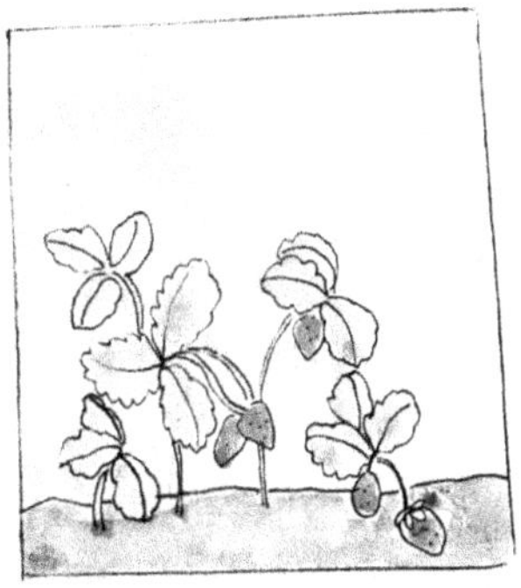

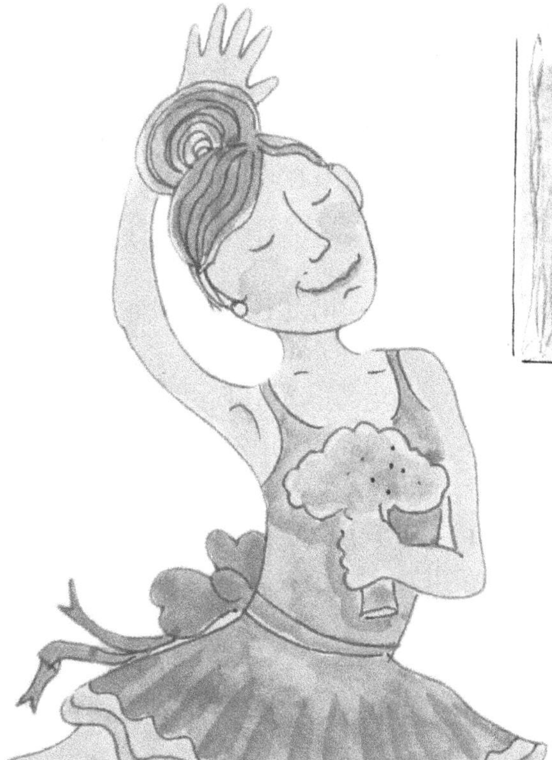

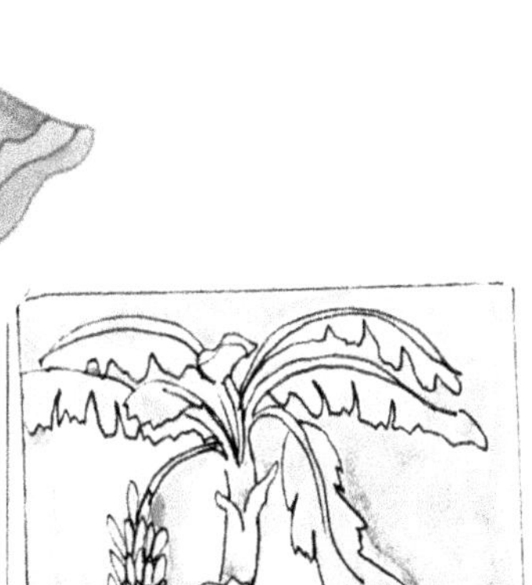

_____

_____

_____

Recipes That Will Delight Your Sweet Tooth

We get used to eating certain foods and enjoying the way they taste. Sometimes, new foods taste a little strange at first, but that is because we have not developed a flavor for them. You see, there are tiny bumps all over our tongue called taste buds. Those bumps allow us to taste things that are sweet, salty, sour, and bitter. We tend to eat the flavors we like. The good news is that our taste buds can change. For example, if we eat a lot of super sweet foods, our taste buds get use to super sweet and desire that flavor. When we eat less sweet foods, our taste buds will change and they will get use to having less sweetened foods. In fact, when we finally eat something super sweet again, we may find we don't like it as much as we use too. It may have become too sweet because we changed the flavors our taste buds desire. Be patient! It takes time for our taste buds to change. You may have to try a new food more than once before you begin to enjoy it.

There are many wonderful recipes you can find with whole sources of sugar. Begin to experiment in the kitchen and keep a notebook of your favorite recipes. On the pages that follow, you will find some tried and true favorites to make when you crave something sweet. As you shop for ingredients listed on these pages, please consider:

Peanut butter: Always buy natural peanut butter. Peanuts should be the only ingredient used.

Chocolate: Buy dark chocolate. Sugar should be listed as one of the last ingredients. If you find chocolate that has been sweetened using stevia, try it! You may like it.

Yogurt: Check labels for sugar! Try buying plain yogurt and get in the habit of sweetening your own yogurt. Most likely you will never use as much sugar as store bought pre-sweetened yogurt.

Maple Syrup: Be sure to buy the real deal 100% maple syrup and not the imitation stuff.

Best Ever Banana Bread

Makes one 9 inch loaf
Ingredients:
4 very ripe bananas
6 tablespoons melted butter
1/3 cup maple syrup
1 egg
2 teaspoons vanilla extract
1 teaspoon baking soda
1/2 teaspoon salt
1 teaspoon cinnamon
1 teaspoon ginger
1 1/2 cups whole wheat pastry flour

MAKE IT:
Preheat oven to 350. Grease a 9 inch bread pan. Mash bananas in a large bowl. Add the rest of the ingredients into the bowl and mix well. Once mixture is well combined pour into greased bread pan. Bake for 50 – 55 min.

*As an extra treat, add a spoonful of maple whipped cream on your bread - see recipe on page 12

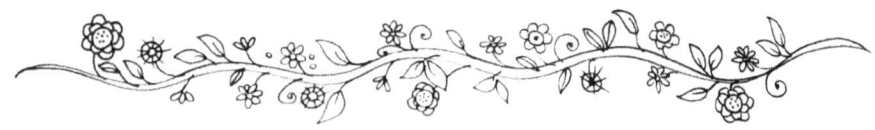

Baked Blueberry Oatmeal Bars with Maple Whipped Cream

Makes 15 bars
Ingredients:
(for baked blueberry oatmeal bars)
1/2 cup coconut oil
3/4 cup maple syrup
2 eggs
2 teaspoons salt
3 1/2 cups quick oats
1 cup coconut milk
1/2 cup dried blueberries (or your favorite choice of fruit)

(for maple whipped cream)
1 cup heavy whipping cream
3 tablespoons maple syrup

MAKE IT:
Preheat oven to 350. Grease an 8 X 11 glass baking dish.

Mix all the ingredients for the oatmeal bars in a large bowl. Once mixture is well combined, pour into prepared baking dish. Bake for 30 min.

While dish is baking make the whipped cream:
Pour 1 cup of heavy whipping cream into a bowl. With an electric mixer, whip the cream on medium speed. Drizzle in maple syrup as you continue to whip. Move to a higher speed until a soft peak has formed. Use whipped cream right away or store in refrigerator.

To Serve: Take one cut bar and place on dish. Spoon a dollop of whipped cream on the baked blueberry oatmeal bar. Delish!

Sweet Parfait

Makes 4 parfaits
Ingredients:
2 cups heavy whipping cream
5 tablespoons honey
10 - 12 strawberries
2 cups granola (see page 17 for recipe)

MAKE IT:
Clean and slice strawberries. Set aside.

Pour 2 cups of heavy whipping cream into a bowl. With an electric mixer, whip the cream on medium speed. Drizzle in honey as you continue to whip. Move to a higher speed until a soft peak has formed. (Use whipped cream right away or store in refrigerator.)

To assemble parfait: Take about five spoonfuls of whipped cream and place in glass. Layer with about five spoonfuls granola. Add another layer of whipped cream. Add a layer of sliced strawberries. Add one more layer of whipped cream. Top with a sprinkle of granola.

Oatmeal Chip Cookies

Makes 24 small cookies
Ingredients:
1 cup quick oats
3/4 cup whole wheat pastry flour
1 1/2 teaspoon baking powder
1 teaspoon cinnamon
1/4 teaspoon salt
1 tablespoon chia seeds
2 tablespoons melted coconut oil
1 egg
2 teaspoons vanilla
1/2 cup honey
1/4 cup mini dark chocolate chips (or take a dark chocolate bar and cut into small chunks)

MAKE IT:
In a medium bowl mix dry ingredients (quick oats, flour, baking powder, cinnamon, salt, chia seeds). In a different medium sized bowl, mix together wet ingredients (coconut oil, egg, vanilla, honey). Add the dry mixture to the wet mixture. Stir until combined. Add in the chocolate chips and stir until even mixed. Chill dough in fridge for about 20 min.

Preheat oven to 350. Line a baking sheet with parchment paper. Spoon 1 inch balls of dough onto prepared cookie sheet (a cookie scoop works great). Bake for 10 - 12 minutes or until cookie is lightly browned. Let cookie cool completely before serving.

Strawberry Yogurt Pops

Makes 12 -15 pops
Ingredients:
1 cup plain yogurt
2 cups sliced strawberries
1 can coconut milk
3 tablespoons honey

popsicle molds
popsicle sticks

MAKE IT:
Place all ingredients in a blender. Blend until smooth. Pour into ice pop molds (small 3oz paper cups work just fine).

Freeze for about 30 min. Add popsicle sticks. Continue to freeze for 2-3 hours. Once the yogurt pop is completely frozen, dig in!

Almond Coconut Bites

Makes 24 bites
Ingredients
1/2 cup coconut butter
1/2 cup almond butter
2 T maple syrup
1 1/2 tablespoons coconut oil
1/2 tsp almond extract
1/2 tsp vanilla
1/4 tsp salt

mini muffin tin
mini cupcake liners

MAKE IT:
Put all the ingredients into a saucepan over medium heat. Stir until combined. Pour into a lined mini muffin tin. Place in freezer for 2 hours. Once the bites have set, they can be stored in the refrigerator. Note: when left out of the fridge at room temperature too long, they will begin to melt. Keep them chilled!

Maple Granola

Makes 16 servings
Ingredients:
6 cups rolled oats
1 1/2 cups maple syrup
1/4 cup coconut oil
1/2 teaspoon salt
1 tablespoon cinnamon
1 teaspoon ginger
1 1/2 cups almond sliced or chopped
3/4 cup chia seeds

MAKE IT:
Preheat oven to 325.

In a large bowl mix together oats, maple syrup, coconut oil, salt, cinnamon, and ginger. Spread this mixture onto a baking sheet (you will probably need two!). Bake for about 30 min. Remove from oven and stir mixture around to get it evenly browned. Return to oven for another 20 min. Remove from oven and stir in the almonds and chia seeds. Return to oven for another 10 min.

The granola is done when it is golden brown and dry. Let it cool completely. Store in an air tight container.

Mint Brownies

Makes 12 brownies
Ingredients:
1 cup melted butter
1/2 cup honey
1/4 cup maple syrup
1 teaspoon vanilla
2 teaspoons peppermint
2 eggs
1/4 cup cocoa powder
1/4 cup coconut flour
1/2 cup rice flour
1 teaspoon baking soda
1 teaspoon salt
2 teaspoons cinnamon

MAKE IT:
Preheat oven to 325

Combine all ingredients in a bowl with a mixer. Grease an 8X8 pan. Pour mixture into prepared pan and bake 25min.

Brownie is done when sides begin to pull away from pan. Note, it may still look wet when removed from oven. Let brownie set for at least 30 min before serving.

Good Morning Cookies

Makes 10 – 12 cookies
Ingredients:
3 cups rolled oats*
1 teaspoon salt
2 teaspoon cinnamon
1 teaspoon ginger
1 teaspoon vanilla
1 cup peanut butter (or your favorite nut butter)
1/4 cup maple syrup
2 large bananas, mashed
1/2 cup mini dark chocolate chips

*put the rolled oats in a food processor and quickly blend until they are almost a flour like consistency OR you can use 2 1/2 cups quick oats

MAKE IT:
Pre heat oven to 325

Place parchment paper on a cookie sheet.

Put all the ingredients in a large bowl. Mix until all ingredients are completely combined. Mixture will be sticky.

Pull out 3 tablespoons of dough and form a ball with your hands. Place ball on lined cookie sheet and flatten ball a little to make a cookie shape. The cookie should be about 1/2 in thick. Repeat with all the dough.

Bake for 15 minutes. The cookies are done when the edges are slightly brown. Be sure to not bake too long or the cookies will dry out.

Store cookies in an air tight container for up to one week.

Peanut Butter Honey Balls

Makes 18-20 balls
Ingredients:
1/2 cup all natural peanut butter
1/3 cup honey
1 cup tapioca flour (also called tapioca starch)
1 cup dark chocolate
1 tablespoon coconut oil

MAKE IT:

In a blender, mix the peanut butter, honey and tapioca flour. Put mixture into a large bowl and knead until a dough ball forms. Grab spoonfuls of mixture and roll into one-inch balls.

Next, slowly melt chocolate and coconut oil over medium heat. Keep stirring carefully not to burn the chocolate! Drop one ball at a time into the melted chocolate. Cover ball entirely in chocolate. Place coated ball on a wax lined cookie sheet. Repeat until all balls are covered in chocolate.

Place in freezer for a minimum of 30 minutes. Once chocolate has cooled and set, put balls in an airtight container and store in refrigerator. Yum!

BONUS!
** If you have extra chocolate make chocolate milk! Pour excess melted chocolate into blender with coconut, almond or soy milk. Cheers!

Store cookies in an air tight container for up to one week.

Chocolate Dip

Dark chocolate combined with coconut oil provides a sweet and rich covering for a treat. Prepare your chocolate and then add your favorite fruit or even nuts to the chocolate.

TO MAKE THE CHOCOLATE SAUCE:
1/2 cup dark chocolate
2 tbs coconut oil

Slowly melt the chocolate and coconut oil over medium heat on the stove. Careful not to burn the chocolate!

OPTIONS FOR DIPPING...

Berry Bites

Makes 14-16 bites
Ingredients:
14 - 16 medium strawberries

MAKE IT:
Prepare the strawberries by washing them and cutting off the green part.

Once the chocolate is melted, take the strawberries and drop them in the chocolate. Cover them completely in chocolate. Place them on a tray covered in wax paper.

Chill in fridge for 20min before serving.

Peanut Butter Banana Bites

Makes 10 – 12 bites
2 bananas
6 tablespoons peanut butter

MAKE IT:
Cut the bananas into 1 inch thick slices. Spread peanut butter on one slice of banana and top with another slice of banana – like a sandwich. Take the peanut butter and banana "sandwich" and dunk it in the chocolate. Place them on a tray covered in wax paper.

Chill in fridge for 20min before serving.

Fill Your Plate

Each day we have choice as to how we will fill our plates and feed our minds. Here is a guideline for how to fuel your mind and body for optimal health. Fill in the blanks with some of your favorite foods. Keep adding to this chart as you explore new whole foods you enjoy eating. Refer to this page as you plan your meals.

Happy and Healthy Eating!

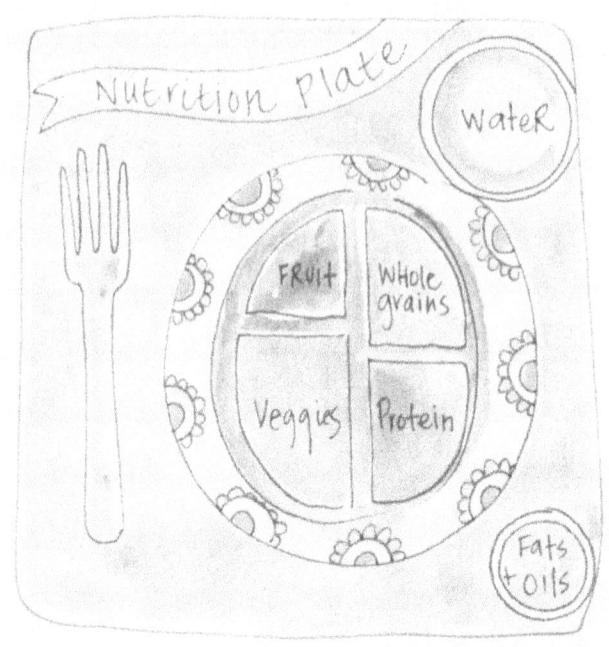

Fruit

_____
_____
_____
_____
_____
_____

Whole Grains

_____
_____
_____
_____
_____
_____

Veggies

_____
_____
_____
_____
_____
_____

Protein

_____
_____
_____
_____
_____
_____

www.ingramcontent.com/pod-product-compliance
Lightning Source LLC
Chambersburg PA
CBHW081352040426
42450CB00015B/3403